NO PRESCRIPTION NEEDED

Living Your Healthiest Life,
Just Ask Your Pharmacist!

DR. GEORGE FRANGIAS

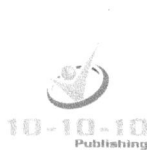

10-10-10
Publishing

No Prescription Needed: Living Your Healthiest Life, Just Ask Your Pharmacist!

www.NoPrescriptionNeededBook.com

Publisher
10-10-10 Publishing
Markham, ON
Canada

Printed in Canada and the United States of America

This book is dedicated to the pharmacists who practice all around the world. I applaud you for all you do to make other peoples lives that much better.

Also, this book is dedicated to my incredible parents, Gerassimos and Stamatia, who are my greatest teachers.

TABLE OF CONTENTS

ACKNOWLEDGMENTS

This book is dedicated to my parents, **Gerassimos and Stamatia Frangias**. Not only would I not be a pharmacist, but I would not be the human being I am today without them. They have supported me financially, emotionally, spiritually, and in so many other ways that I can't possibly list it all without writing a whole other book about it! I continue to remain grateful for the love and support they give to me every single day. They deeply inspire with their work ethic and devotion to their family and loved ones. I want to extend a special thanks and gratitude to my siblings—**Andreas, Angie, and Basil**—for their continued support and love. (**Basil**, an extra thank you for being one of the main catalysts on my personal growth journey, which has had a powerful impact, not only on my practice but on every aspect of my life. For that, I will always be grateful.)

Raymond Aaron

From the bottom of my heart, thank you for being my teacher, mentor and friend. Your impact on my life has been so uplifting and inspirational, that I can't express my gratitude enough! This book wouldn't have become a reality without you. I look forward to my continued growth with your guidance.

Professor John Papastergiou

A personal thank you to Professor John Papastergiou, RPh., my mentor and friend. Being awarded the OPA Mentorship Award, and named Canadian Pharmacist of the Year, your work in research and community practice is being recognized and inspiring internationally. In 2019, being named by the International Forum on Advancement in Healthcare, as one of the top 100 healthcare leaders globally, was certainly something to celebrate. Your dedication to your patients, and to the Pharmacy profession as a whole, constantly encourages and inspires me.

Dr Maria Psihogios

Thank you for displaying the compassion and presence you show in your practice and as a human being every day of your life. You are a shining example of what doctors and people can strive to become. May you continue to inspire others as much as you inspire me to continue to grow.

The Canadian Pharmacists Association

Advancing the health and well-being of Canadians through excellence in pharmacist care is exactly what the Canadian Pharmacist Association (CPhA) does. Your vision of "pharmacists providing world-class pharmacy leadership" is something I live by. I am very proud to be a part of this association, because we really are "stronger together."

Ontario College of Pharmacists

Thank you to the Ontario College of Pharmacists (OCP) for continuing to serve and protect the public. I have devoted my life to serving the public, and sharing the mandate of the OCP is very important to me. I am grateful for the guidance, knowledge, and resources in making pharmacists the best they can be in order to deliver the best care possible.

Ontario Pharmacists Association

Many thanks to the Ontario Pharmacists Association (OPA) for advocating excellence in practice and patient care. Whatever a pharmacist or pharmacy needs, you are there to offer unending support. The OPA is usually the first place I call when I need help in my practice, whether it is patient specific or pharmacy operations related, and you always have answers I seek. Thank you for advancing the Pharmacy profession as a vital healthcare provider, through advocacy, innovation, and support services.

OnPharm-United

A special thank you to OnPharm-United for being committed to strengthening independent pharmacy owners to help their business and practice thrive through leveraging the network's programs, resources, and strategic partnerships. It is no surprise that pharmacies continue to join in a shared vision for the profession, and your support is greatly appreciated.

Canadian Foundation for Pharmacy

Since 1945, the Canadian Foundation for Pharmacy has been helping countless individuals and organizations, while achieving its mandate to advance the profession of Pharmacy. Thank you for being a leader in pharmacy evolution and innovation.

The Neighbourhood Pharmacy Association of Canada

Thank you to The Neighbourhood Pharmacy Association of Canada for being focused on the business of neighbourhood pharmacy, ensuring that independent pharmacies can continue to deliver the convenient, professional patient care products and services on which Canadians rely.

Massachusetts College of Pharmacy

One of the happiest days of my life was the day I received my Doctorate in Pharmacy (PharmD) degree from Massachusetts

College of Pharmacy and Health Sciences (MCPHS), in the distinguished city of Boston, MA, in the USA. It was truly a defining moment in my life when I successfully completed my 6-year Pharmacy program, which gave me the knowledge and tools to start my Pharmacy practice. Thank you to Charles F. Monahan, then president of MCPHS, for his dedication to ensuring the high standards of quality I experienced while attending. Also, a special thank you to Paul DiFrancesco, Associate Dean of Pharmacy Experiential Education, who personally assured me that everything was going to work out, while I was going through a struggle during my schooling and wasn't so sure.

University of Toronto

Even though my time was brief at the University of Toronto (UofT), it was where I started my journey toward becoming a pharmacist. I learned some tough lessons during my time at UofT, which only helped me grow that much faster. UofT has evolved into Canada's leading institution of learning, discovery, and knowledge creation. I feel very privileged that I had the opportunity to learn at such a historic institution.

University of Waterloo

Thank you to the University of Waterloo for being just the second School of Pharmacy in the great province of Ontario, Canada. You have created more opportunities for individuals to join this rewarding Pharmacy profession.

I wish to extend great thanks to **The Right Honourable Justin Trudeau**, Prime Minister of Canada. Canada's healthcare system is one that many other countries strive to duplicate. I am honoured to be a part of this great institution that is continually being improved upon. Thank you to **Doug Ford**, Premier of Ontario, for continuing this province's dedication to outstanding healthcare. Also, thank you to the mayor of the city I was born and raised in, and currently practice Pharmacy in, **John Tory**, Mayor of Toronto. Many thanks to you and your office for helping Torontonians continue to receive the healthcare they deserve.

Thank you **CBC, CTV, Global News, CityTV, TVOntario, Toronto Star, Toronto Sun,** and to the many other local and national news outlets that keep the public up to date on timely information that can concern their health and well-being. Their assistance with healthcare promotion and notification is extremely important for the public's health and safety.

FOREWORD

W hen you think of a pharmacist, do you think of just another healthcare professional in a white coat? Perhaps someone to simply dispense your prescription or give you advice on which cold medication you should take? Perhaps you are a pharmacist yourself, and need a boost to your outlook and spirit when it comes to your career.

Written from a pharmacist's perspective, *No Prescription Needed* will help shine some light on how valuable pharmacy and pharmacists can be in your health journey. If you are already a pharmacist, it will reignite the passion for your profession, and help you remember why you wanted to become a pharmacist in the first place: to help others!

Even if you aren't a pharmacist and happen to come upon this book, you will gain a full scope of how a pharmacist fits into your health care team. It will also empower you to seek out your pharmacist for a new type of relationship, and begin really including him or her as part of your health care team. This book is an invaluable tool in understanding who a pharmacist is, everything they can and already are doing, and the great potential the profession has.

I have had the pleasure of getting to know Dr. George Frangias ever since he started on his personal development journey by attending a class of mine in 2018. I am inspired by George's patient and community-based approach to his work, and how he handles his practice. Year after year, it is no wonder that he continues to find success. Working as a pharmacist is George's greatest passion. His knowledge, expertise and commitment to growth are admirable. Not only does he keep up to date with everything "pharmacy," but his devotion to personal development outside pharmacy is constantly improving his practice, and himself as a human being. No doubt you will be inspired to regain control of your health, or to follow in his footsteps when establishing your own business. You may even want to reach out to him directly to talk about how you can level up your own practice, and your approach to your work.

—**Raymond Aaron**
New York Times Bestselling Author

Chapter 1

CHOOSING MY LIFE'S WORK

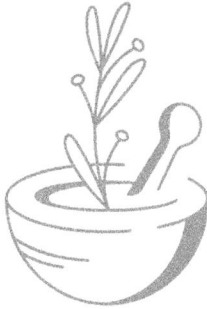

*"Be kind,
for everyone you meet
is fighting a hard battle."*

–Plato

1

As a child, I never dreamed of being a pharmacist. I didn't even know what a pharmacist was or what they actually did until I got my first job as a teenager. My upbringing was pretty typical for a child of immigrant parents. My parents moved from Greece to Toronto in hopes of creating a better future for themselves. While my father worked in the restaurant industry 6 (sometimes 7) days a week, my mother stayed home and took care of the children. (I was the second oldest of four kids.) We lived modestly but, all things considered, actually had all we needed growing up. I can see how hard my parents worked to ensure that we were well taken care of and surrounded with love. We were a typical and traditional Greek family living in the city, and this instilled a deep sense of pride for my heritage that I still hold close today. I want to honor and stay connected to my roots, while at the same time feeling so blessed and grateful to be living in such a great country.

When I reflect back on it, being an academic wasn't really where I started. Maybe it was because I was just a kid and interested in other things. I can remember a turning point for me though. It came in grade 5 when I was tired of cheating off someone else in math class. Up until that point I didn't have a strong relationship to learning or what that meant to me. However, after it hit me that I couldn't continue this way, something inside me said "Enough is enough" and I began taking my schooling very seriously. From that point on I was consistently in the higher-grade average in my class, especially when it came to math and sciences, all through elementary school and highschool. I am grateful as this gave me the strong foundation I needed for my career.

When I was 16, I wanted to gain some independence by having my own source of income, as many teenagers do. Within walking distance of my home was a family owned and operated pharmacy. Doug, the owner, gave me a break and offered me my first part time job as a "stock boy" for their business. I spent two nights a week at the pharmacy stocking shelves and getting to know the owner and staff as well. We got along really well and soon enough he offered me a promotion to work the front cash. This is where I really began seeing and understanding the role of a pharmacist in the community. I watched as people came in and out of the pharmacy, day after day, getting prescriptions filled or picking up personal health products for themselves and their families. By working at the cash, I began gaining an appreciation for who was frequenting the pharmacy and why. Some customers I began seeing regularly, and some only once in a while. But I could tell that the pharmacy was an essential part of my community.

After a year and a half of working there, the owner could see that my interest and involvement in the business was strong. Again, I was offered a promotion, this time to pharmacy assistant. This was so exciting for me! I went from working up at the front of the pharmacy at the cash to working side by side with the pharmacist. This is where my understanding of *exactly* what a pharmacist does, and how they are essential health care providers within a community, became clearer. Day in and day out, I worked alongside the pharmacist and gained insight into why the pharmacist and customer relationship is so important. This wasn't just about getting prescriptions filled. This was about being on the front line of the patient's well-being. It was the bridge between a diagnosis and a plan of care.

I will never forget one encounter that literally changed my life. One afternoon, we were working as usual, when an elderly woman approached the counter with tears running down her face. At first, I thought she was upset at the pharmacist, and that we had done something to harm her. I thought she was angry and was coming in to give us a piece of her mind. However, as the conversation unfolded, I realized she was crying tears of joy! She had specifically come in to offer sincere thanks to the pharmacist to how good she was feeling. I learned that the pharmacist had been in touch with her doctor and advocated that she be taken *off* a few medications that he felt she no longer needed to be on. Several weeks after stopping those medications, her health had improved so dramatically that she was able to leave her bed, where she had spent most of her time feeling sick. Now she was feeling the best she had in a long time, and it was thanks to the pharmacist. She expressed how she felt she had been given her life back. I was so extremely moved by this encounter that it became clear to me that I wanted to help others live their best lives, as the pharmacist had. I wanted to be an advocate for patients and help them lead healthy and happy lives, full of energy and inspiration. From that point on, I had decided I would go to school to become a pharmacist in order to be part of my community in a meaningful and life changing way.

In this book I want to explore with you the field of Pharmacy and the role a pharmacist plays in your life. In my experience, when it comes down to it, pharmacists aren't always given the respect they deserve. Whether you are a patient, a student or in the healthcare industry, I know this book will provide you with some key knowledge and understanding as to how a pharmacist fits into your health care team. We are here for you and always ready to open a dialogue about your health or the health of a loved one. If you are a patient I want you to know you can always talk to your pharmacist, **no prescription needed!** Let's start at the beginning and learn about how Pharmacy started and grew into the extensive field it is today.

Chapter Summary

- You never know where you will find your life's passion.

- Mentorship can create change and excite the new generation

- Clear and open communication between a Pharmacist and their patient can change lives for the better

- Pharmacists are key members of your health care team that deserve more respect than they are generally given

Chapter 2

THE HISTORY OF PHARMACY

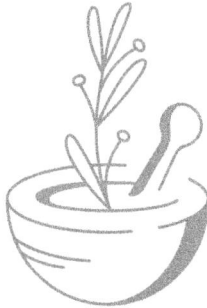

"Medicine is not only a science; it is also an art. It does not consist of compounding pills and plasters; it deals with the very processes of life, which must be understood before they may be guided."

–Paracelsus

2

D o you really understand what *Pharmacy* is? Or what your pharmacist really does besides dispensing your prescription given to you by your healthcare prescriber?

Pharmacy can be thought of as a science *and* an art! It focuses on the preparation and the standardization of medications available with a prescription, and over-the-counter medications that do not require one. Pharmacy practices have some of their roots dating as far back as in ancient Greece. Of course, it looked a lot different then! The roots of pharmacy practices lie in acts such as extracting juices and oils from plants and using them as an aid to healing the body. In history, there were two distinct classes of physicians: One would visit the sick, and one would make the remedies to aid the sick. This is where the distinction between physician and pharmacist began.

You can see that in ancient Greece, Rome, and then in Europe through the middle ages, the healing arts were clearly defined between the physician doctor and the herbalist. Around 400 BC, some of the best known early practitioners/ pharmacists were recorded. One example is Diocles of Carystus, who was a Greek member of the "rhizotomoi," a specialized branch of medical experts on the uses of medicinal plants. Then during 50–70 AD, Pedanius Dioscorides, a Greek physician in the Roman army, wrote a five-volume book entitled, *De Materia Medica,* meaning *"concerning medicinal substances or on medical material."* This became THE book on medicinal plants, and was recognized as the main source of pharmaceutical medicine for 1500 years!

Again, it was the physician who understood the patients' ailments, and then the herbalist was the one creating or preparing the "medicine," so to speak. However, the Arabian influence in Europe, during the 8th century AD, really began to solidify the two roles as two separate professions. From there, pivotal moments in the history of pharmaceutical medicine came. These events created the cornerstones for the modern distinction of the role of a pharmacist as we know it today.

An example of these dramatic changes can be seen in 1683, when the city of Bruges (Belgium) forbade physicians to prepare their own medicine. This helped reinforce the expectations and different duties performed by physicians and pharmacists. It helped create some distinguishing factors for each, and highlight how they each are a specialist in what they do. At the end of the day this would only benefit the patient because where only one healthcare practitioner was used, there would now be two, thus creating more focus and a possibility of personalized care.

We can then go on to see another major transition in how Pharmacy branches out to become more of an independent industry in 1751 when Benjamin Franklin helped establish the Pennsylvania Hospital (USA). Not only was this the first public hospital in North America, it also housed the first established in-hospital pharmacy. At the time, according to city leaders of the Philadelphia region, there was deep concern for public health on the whole as they recognized an uptick of general infections and diseases. So Benjamin Franklin, along with Dr. Thomas Bond, founded the hospital, making a commitment to not only take care of the community from a physical health perspective but also from a mental health perspective.

After World War II, the pharmaceutical industry took on some dramatic changes. The needs of the industry changed, and the role of the pharmacist changed as well. Pharmacists were no longer required to be truly involved in the preparation of the medicine. Before this, pharmacists were still responsible for the actual preparation of pills, potions, etc. Medications were beginning to be manufactured, so the pharmacist's focus changed to solely storing and dispensing medications, giving advice, and assuring that the well-being of patients be a priority.

The Pharmacist Today

"Healthy citizens are the greatest asset any country can have."
–Winston Churchill

The role of a pharmacist, today, is becoming more and more like that of a physician, in a sense. Like discussing health concerns with a physician, oftentimes, we sit down with our patients to assess and offer advice, as opposed to just standing behind a counter and handing off medications. A bonus is that the patient does not need an appointment to talk to us. They can just walk up to the counter and ask for help: **No prescription needed!**

Pharmacists are equipped to assess minor conditions such as seasonal allergies and skin irritations, to name a few. This can be a highly beneficial situation for the patient, as they will be able to seek relief immediately for what is ailing them—and it beats waiting at the walk-in clinic or having to wait weeks to see your doctor! Patients can see their pharmacist to get their "flu shot" (flu vaccine), as well as other travel vaccines and injections. In your busy day-to-day lives, it is incredible to think that you now have the option to do this. It is very convenient and offers people so much value.

This convenience even extends further! Patients can also go to their pharmacist for advice on how to live a healthier lifestyle. For example, if you wanted to quit smoking, you could talk to your pharmacist about different ways you could be supported during that time. If your pharmacist chooses to, they can prescribe medication right on the spot to help you start your smoke-free journey. Each time I help someone start the journey to quitting smoking it really does bring me such joy! From a medical standpoint the change in your body, even just within the first hour, is remarkable. For example, within 8 hours, oxygen levels in your blood return to normal and the levels of nicotine and carbon monoxide are reduced by more than half. Then looking ahead to being 24 hours smoke free, carbon monoxide has been fully eliminated from your body and your lungs begin the process of detoxing. I use the example of helping a patient quit smoking as a powerful reminder of how your pharmacist can be of service to your health in the most immediate of ways. Also personally, it is something that springs to mind as I always love celebrating when my patients are ready to make some large personal shifts such as quitting smoking. I always feel so proud of them and grateful they are willing to create change.

Pharmacists are also equipped to support you in managing chronic diseases (e.g., asthma, chronic pain, etc.) by offering education and advice. This can include a range of things such as advising on how to properly use asthma puffers with beneficial attachments like a "spacer" (with or without a mask) to ensure the medication ends up in your lungs and not just on the back of your throat. They can also recommend which puffer is best for you according to your severity. By delivering the medication to your lungs properly, unnecessary dose increases can be avoided in instances where the patient and/or prescriber might have thought too low of a dose was being used. When it comes to chronic pain, pharmacists are well equipped to offer immediate support to a patient. From positioning the painful area of the body at a certain level, using braces and supports to recommending topical remedies (creams, ointments, gels), and what medication is best based on the level of swelling. A pharmacist can help individualize a treatment plan specific to each patient. All of this may be taken advantage of all under one roof and sometimes without having to ever leave the neighborhood!

Pharmacists are an incredible, local resource to the community. When you begin to cultivate a relationship and collaborate with your pharmacist, seeing them as an integral part of your health care team (just as much as say your doctor, dentist, and other health care providers you regularly see), your path to living a more vibrant and healthy life will be brighter and easier!

"Health is a state of complete mental, social and physical well-being, not merely the absence of disease or infirmity."
–World Health Organization, 1948

As I mentioned, I have always known that I wanted to pursue a career as a pharmacist. Though, as with many things in life, it wasn't always an easy road to follow. During that period of young adulthood, I had to do a lot of personal growing (and fast!) in order to ensure my dreams would come true.

Chapter Summary

- Pharmacy can be thought of as a science (as well as an art)

- Pharmacy has roots dating back to ancient Greece and Rome

- Pharmacy dramatically changed after WWII with the modernization of producing medications

- Every year pharmacists are taking on more and more roles similar to a physician

- Year after year, a pharmacist will be able to provide more services to a patient, therefore creating more ease and convenience in one's life

- Because of their expertise and personalized care, pharmacists are an indispensable part of the community

Chapter 3

MY ROAD TO BECOMING A PHARMACIST

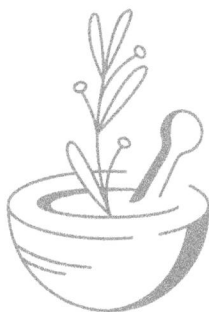

"We must all suffer one of two things: the pain of discipline or the pain of regret. The difference is discipline weighs ounces while regret weighs tons."

– Jim Rohn

3

As I mentioned, after gaining insight into how essential a pharmacist is for personal health care, I knew I wanted to go to school to study Pharmacy. There was no question about it! I felt very confident about starting university, as I had always been a great student. However, I was soon to find out that the path to realizing my dream wasn't going to be as easy as I thought.

During my second year in the Life Sciences program at the University of Toronto, my grades started to dip. They dipped so low in fact, I was suspended. This was a challenging and humiliating setback for me to accept. Out of all my siblings, I was always consistently the best student. Even amongst my peers, I excelled and was known for being academically successful. I didn't understand how this could happen when just a few years earlier, I was valedictorian when graduating junior high school. It was especially hard to get up the courage to tell my parents what had happened! They had previously shared the news with family and friends that I was my junior high school valedictorian, and now I didn't know how I was going to share this news. I felt so nervous and even a bit embarrassed. So much in fact, I can remember the moment so clearly even to this day. One morning, my father was shaving, and I worked up all the courage to tell him the sad news. "Dad, I've been suspended from school." At first, he thought I was joking! He couldn't believe it. Then the reality set in, and he knew it was true. I had temporarily lost the focus required to fulfill my dream of becoming a pharmacist. This lack of focus cost me my place at the university, and the belief that others previously had in me of accomplishing great things, or so I thought. I sat down and had a long talk with my parents about the next steps. We looked at my options and, at this point, with such low grades at U of T (University of Toronto), we knew it was going to be nearly impossible for me to get into Pharmacy school in Toronto, let alone Canada. Admission was very limited at the schools, and competition was fierce. It was decided that I should begin looking into schools in the USA, hoping that this was a possible alternative.

"Divide each difficulty into as many parts as is feasible and necessary to resolve it, and watch the whole transform."

– Rene Descartes

After more research, it was clear that in order to achieve my dream of being a pharmacist, I was going to have to attend a school in the United States. From a logistical standpoint, there were more Pharmacy schools to choose from, so it seemed I would have a better chance of being accepted somewhere. However, one major hurdle, besides having my confidence bruised from my suspension, was the fact that my tuition fees would now be *5 times* the cost compared to a school in Canada (and not to mention in USD). As a young adult, I didn't have that kind of savings at all! My parents were put into a difficult position. How could they afford to send me to school as an international student, especially after getting suspended from university here? Not to mention my three siblings were all close in age and still in post secondary studies themselves. Yes, I had been suspended due to low grades, but they could see my renewed passion and drive for my path to being a pharmacist and helping people. Even my family doctor independently advocated for me to go to the States. He assured my parents that sending me to pharmacy school in the USA would end up being the best investment they could make. I was very touched to have him in my court.

I began applying for schools, and my parents said they would figure out finances when the time came, based on whether I got into a Pharmacy program at all. Thankfully, I was accepted into Massachusetts College of Pharmacy and Health Sciences (MCPHS), in Boston, Massachusetts. It just so happened to be the same college that my employer at the pharmacy (Doug), and his brother (Steve), went to many years before. I looked at this coincidence as a sign that I was on the right path again! A door had once again opened to realizing my dream of becoming a pharmacist. Along with being accepted, I also received the news that I had been awarded a scholarship of $7500, based on my academic achievement in high school. Amazing! I was accepted into several different Pharmacy schools in the US; however, at the end of the day, everything pointed toward attending MCPHS.

With this new opportunity before me, my parents continued to have faith in me. Then MCPHS hit us with a roadblock. Not only would I have to provide documents that I could afford the $25,000 USD (after subtracting the $7500 scholarship) tuition for the first year, but also proof that I would be able to continue to cover the tuition for each consecutive year in the six-year PharmD program. It was in this situation that my parents truly came to my rescue. They expressed that they had such faith in me that they were willing to take a loan out for my tuition, using our family home as collateral. With that loan, I was able to show the school that tuition would not be a problem during the six years, and I was invited to attend. Wow… I still feel immense gratitude toward them and the lengths they were willing to go to in order to help me follow my path.

During my 6 years at MCPHS, I lived on campus for 5 of them: my first year as a freshman with suitemates, two years as a Resident Assistant, and then taking on the role of Head Resident Assistant for the last two years. During my time as Head Resident Assistant, I was given the opportunity to practice my passion for helping others! Not only was I someone the residents on my floor could come to for information and guidance regarding the Pharmacy program and living on campus, but like a pharmacist, I had to be ready to help solve any problems they had. I helped students through things like managing stress, to interpersonal relations, to even how to remain happy and positive while being away from home. I felt in my element and part of a bigger picture for the residents on my floor. I acted as a leader in the community we created, and I loved it. It was an invaluable learning experience for what was waiting for me after graduation.

After six intense and incredible years at MCPHS, I received my Doctorate in Pharmacy. One of the proudest moments in my life was going up on stage to receive my diploma, looking out into the audience, and seeing my parents and sister cheering me on. It was such an incredible feeling, which I will never forget! As I looked out over the audience, I had flashbacks of the suspension from U of T, the embarrassment I felt, having to move to a different country for school and taking on the responsibility of knowing that our family's house was on the line for me to succeed. In that moment of overwhelming joy and accomplishment, all of that stress and pressure lifted off my shoulders, and I knew that a new chapter of my life was ready to begin.

"A good laugh and a long sleep are the best cures in the doctor's book."
- Irish proverb

I was looking forward to returning to Toronto to take my licensing tests so that I may start practicing being a pharmacist in my community. There is a written component and an in-person practical component to become licensed as a pharmacist. I passed the practical component, which involved entering a bunch of exam rooms where there was an evaluator playing a patient with an issue you had to try and solve in a short period of time. As stressful as this was,

I passed this on my first attempt and felt so relieved. This sense of accomplishment and relief didn't last long. Another obstacle quickly appeared though. This time, I failed the written portion of my exam and had to wait another 6 months in order to rewrite it. I had come so far and could not let this discourage me. So I took the time, worked even harder, and knew I passed the test even before receiving the result! Now, with both my Pharmacy Doctorate and practicing License in hand, I was truly ready to begin my career as a practicing pharmacist.

At this time, in Toronto, finding a full-time position as a pharmacist proved to be challenging. But I was eager to get my feet wet and begin serving my community. I took on a part-time role back at the pharmacy where I worked as a teenager, back in the neighborhood I grew up in (talk about coming full circle!). I also kept an eye out for work as a relief pharmacist covering shifts all over the city, and I even helped out a friend by covering for him at his pharmacy when needed. (Since I was fluent in Greek, I could serve his patients well at a mostly Greek speaking community pharmacy.) I was so hungry for experience that I took any job opportunity that came my way, even flying out of the city to rural parts of the province for short stints. For years, I continued to hit the ground running as hard as I could, bouncing from pharmacy to pharmacy, trying to fill my week.

During this time of jumping from one pharmacy to another, I came to the realization that I would love to have my own pharmacy. I wasn't willing to just wait for a position to open up and hope it would work out. I wanted to be my own boss and directly be responsible for my patients' well-being. I wanted to make my dreams come true on my own terms, as I always had. On October 16, 2017, I purchased an existing pharmacy from a pharmacist that was retiring, and I opened Bloor St Pharmacy, in downtown Toronto. Turning this longstanding pharmacy into a modern, thriving business and health center for the neighborhood, became my number one priority, and I never looked back!

When I look back at the young boy who realized his passion for helping others, to me now, as not only a pharmacist but as a business owner, so many things have changed. But some things have always remained true: my drive, my willingness to do what it takes to achieve my goals, and my absolute passion to be part of people's health care teams. I truly want my patients to be leading their best life, and I am so grateful that I have set myself up where I can do that. I also have deep gratitude for my struggles, as it puts me in a position to provide mentorship and be a leader for other aspiring pharmacists. If you want something bad enough, you can absolutely make your dreams come true.

Let's dive back into discussing more in detail the role of a pharmacist and some particulars of their work, and let's begin with taking a look at the different environments you may find a pharmacist in (some of which may surprise you!).

Chapter Summary

- The transition from secondary to post secondary education can be extremely difficult and challenging, but there is always a way to find your way back to your path

- When on your path to achieving your goals, always find a great support system to help you along the way (especially in rocky times!)

- It's important to connect to what you really love about what you are studying and hone in on the possibilities that may be offered (For myself, it was the possibility of opening my own pharmacy so that I may stay as close to the community as possible)

Chapter 4

DIFFERENT ENVIRONMENTS PHARMACISTS WORK IN

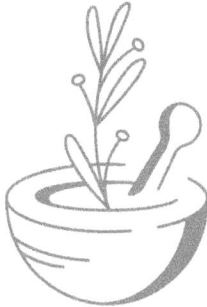

"Our bodies are our gardens; our wills are our gardeners."

–William Shakespeare

4

When you picture a pharmacist, the first image that probably comes to mind is your local neighborhood pharmacist. You see them behind the counter at your local pharmacy, most likely wearing a white coat and either filling your prescription or giving you advice on some over-the-counter medication, be it a supplement for general health or something that may help with symptoms you are experiencing. However, what you may not know is that pharmacists are found in many different environments and different roles. You will find them in patient-centered environments or non-patient environments. Let's specifically examine some of them. (And for those in the field of Pharmacy, or those wanting to be, I urge you to open your mind and pay close attention!)

Patient-Centered Environments

"There is one consolation in being sick; and that is the possibility that you may recover to a better state than you were ever in before."

–Henry David Thoreau

There are several distinct patient-centered environments that pharmacists will be found working in. Obviously the main point of focus here is the direct relationship to the patient. When working in a patient-centered environment, the pharmacist is presented with the opportunity to really get up close and personal with people. Some may thrive in these sorts of environments, some may not. It is important, especially if you are just starting a career in pharmacy to understand where your strengths lie and if working directly with patients one on one is for you. It requires a particular mindset and level of interpersonal skills. (There is no shame if your strengths do not lie here as there are numerous other opportunities which I will touch on later.)

One of the main environments that you are familiar with, as mentioned above, are community pharmacies or what is also referred to as a retail pharmacy. These environments serve the public directly and, as indicated, are located right in the heart of communities. For example, my current practice is considered a community pharmacy. These are amazing hubs of wellness and health. A community pharmacy can be seen as the cornerstone of many people's plans of care for maintaining a healthy lifestyle or any illness, ranging from something acute/short-term like treating a cold/flu, or if they are dealing with a more long-term or chronic illness like rheumatoid arthritis. They will constantly be coming in and out to get prescriptions filled, or picking up health products to make their lives even healthier. When you work as a pharmacist at a community-based practice, it is an incredible opportunity to really create deep and personal relationships with people. A pharmacist can really get to know someone's health history and, therefore, be able to provide them with the best care possible. As a pharmacist, not only will you be getting to know your patients, you will also be interacting with other healthcare professionals, such as family physicians, specialists, naturopathic doctors, psychiatrists, dentists, nurse practitioners, optometrists, registered nurses, medical and nursing assistants, therapists, veterinarians, and other pharmacists and pharmacy technicians, just to name a few! Imagine the possibilities of growth for the pharmacist and the pharmacy when in this sort of environment!

Pharmacists can also be found outside the pharmacy, with their own office in medical buildings as part of a family health team. These are also health and wellness hubs that serve all ages, and a place where whole families may go together. This presents an amazing opportunity to really get to know families, their health histories, and lifestyles as a whole. That kind of knowledge is very powerful. In these family health teams, pharmacists will work alongside doctors, nurses, and other healthcare practitioners as part of a team. Pharmacists oversee anything medication-related. They also take the lead in educating other team members on current evidence-based medication treatments, as well as new options that may become available for patients. This is a crucial role to play so that the whole health professional team can be on the same page as to what can be best for the patients, and be up to date on how a patient can be helped most effectively.

Another patient-centered environment is a hospital. Pharmacists here will either work with "in-patients" (those who are admitted to the hospital and can stay overnight) or with "out-patients" (those who come in for an appointment to see their doctor or specialist, and then leave to go back home). A hospital can definitely be a fast-paced environment where there is constantly a flow of patients in and out of the building. A pharmacist's role may also be seen as being of the utmost importance by patients and their loved ones, as you will be recommending and providing medication that may even be saving someone's life, depending on the severity of the situation.

One patient-centered environment that many forget about are long-term care and assisted-living facilities. In these special environments, you may actually be seen as part of someone's extended family, as these patients are actually living together. These spaces can be very intimate and very rewarding to work in depending on your personality.

Pharmacists are even found in the Armed Forces. What a distinctive opportunity! When working with the military department of the federal government, you may work directly with soldiers and doctors to provide injury treatment, emergency medicine, and intensive-care therapy. This kind of care may take place at a military base or a field medical unit. Here, pharmacists would be required to meet the strong mental and physical health standards, like all other members of the armed forces, on top of the usual pharmacist qualifications. This would be a unique and deeply fulfilling opportunity for a specific kind of person, no doubt!

Non-Patient-Centered Environments

"It is health that is the real wealth, and not pieces of gold and silver."

–Mahatma Gandhi

There are opportunities for pharmacists to also work in environments where there isn't necessarily a lot, if any, patient interaction. These positions are just as important though, and depending on your strengths, it may even suit one better! I have many colleagues that are thriving in these non-patient-centered environments, whereas I thrive in my community-based practice. It is important to understand that there are opportunities for everyone, no matter where you feel you can contribute most; and as a pharmacist, you can find many opportunities for work, beyond working behind a counter dispensing medications.

One of the first places to consider applying yourself as a pharmacist is working in a university or college environment. As professors, pharmacists help develop the next generation that will play integral roles in their communities. There are opportunities to teach full-term classes or act as a special guest speaker, perhaps specializing in something you are passionate about or identify as an expert in. The possibility of speaking at a post- secondary institution can also be looked at as something you may pursue on the side of working in a pharmacy or a hospital. You can definitely create some of your own opportunities here. Because you will be researching and preparing material to pass on to eager minds, teaching is a great way to stay up to date with the latest in the pharmacy world. At the same time, you will have the opportunity to offer your students an insight to real life application from your actual practice in the community.

The government also has opportunities for pharmacists in the way of research and being a consultant. Governments have their own medical boards and sectors, which pharmacists are definitely called upon in terms of lending their expertise and professional opinion. Clear examples are during the SARS and Covid-19 outbreaks, to name a few recent ones. So many health care experts were needed for these outbreaks to be contained and resolved. When working directly in the Government, Pharmacists are given the opportunity to play their roles as medication experts, and to contribute to resolving these particular stressful and serious situations.

In usual day to day business, pharmacists involved in government can aid officials in making informed decisions when looking at public health care and also legislature.

Pharmaceutical companies will obviously employ dozens of pharmacists. These pharmacists will work alongside doctors, scientists, and other medical researchers in many different arenas. There is research and development of new drugs, clinical trials, and further development of existing drugs. It is essential for pharmacists to be key players at pharmaceutical companies, as they will eventually be looked to as the experts of the products that the companies are developing. This type of position can be very exciting for someone who thrives on working on teams, and excels in research-based work. For example, pharmacists were some of the many experts involved in seeing if the medication *hydroxychloroquine* (traditionally used for malaria and rheumatoid arthritis) would be effective or not in the treatment for Covid-19 infected patients. While some countries reported this treatment to be effective against Covid-19, and other countries not so much, these conclusions wouldn't have been possible without the assistance of pharmacists. Pharmacists bring their understanding to existing medications and side effects when testing new drugs, which is essential when analyzing test results and patient symptoms. This can be seen as yet another example of how a pharmacist and physician truly work side by side in health care.

I'm sure this has once again opened your mind to the possibilities that can lie ahead for one in the field of Pharmacy. It excited me when I began learning about all the opportunities available to me, and the different avenues that I could pursue. On my own path, I just always came back to what led me into the field of Pharmacy, and it was always clear to me what environment I wanted to be in. Who knows what the future has in store for me, and I can't wait to find out!

Let's continue to explore these different avenues, focusing on the different services a pharmacist may offer, again demonstrating the vast array of contributions a pharmacist can make in the field of health care.

Chapter Summary

- Pharmacists work in several different environments, beyond just the pharmacy counter which patients may be most familiar with

- Pharmacists also work in medical buildings, hospitals and long-term care facilities

- The Army also has pharmacists on staff to assist in operations

- Pharmacists will often work in University or College environments as professors to teach and inspire a new generation

- You will also find roles for pharmacists in governments and pharmaceutical companies (with focuses on research and development respectively)

Chapter 5

SERVICES OFFERED BY PHARMACISTS

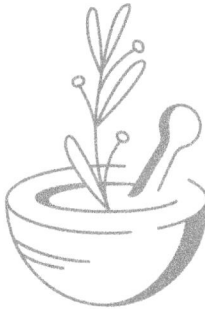

"Give a man health and a course to steer, and he'll never stop to trouble about whether he's happy or not."

– George Bernard Shaw

5

As we continue to cover the in's and out's of how a pharmacist fits into the health care picture, I want to now thoroughly discuss specific services provided by a pharmacist. Some of these services you may be aware of; however, I bet there are a few services that you didn't realize a pharmacist could assist you with! (Please keep in mind that some are depending on province or state, or even country as well.)

Managing Medication Profiles

Perhaps you know someone who is currently dealing with a lot of health issues, or even perhaps you yourself are juggling many health concerns. It is possible for someone to take many medications at once to treat a multitude of symptoms and illnesses. However, you have to be mindful and aware that medications sometimes cannot be taken together or even at certain times in your day. This is where a pharmacist can come in and assist you in managing these medications. You don't have to do all the work in sorting through instructions and adverse reaction warnings. Nor should you be expected to. Allow your pharmacist to do this for you! Pharmacists are able to provide insight into

41

medications, their potential side effects, resulting drug interactions, and much more.

Serious drug interactions can be an issue if you are taking multiple medications at a time. Sometimes you have to start taking a medication while already on another, or perhaps you have to take different ones at different times. It must be taken seriously as drug interactions can result in adverse (negative) reactions, even a trip to the emergency room in the direst of situations. Pharmacists are more than happy to work with you to ensure that this doesn't happen and that you stay safe. I have helped multiple patients in ensuring that they don't experience adverse reactions when combining their medications, and even helped some people stop taking some medications that they no longer need, all by simplifying their medication regimen. Of course, this was after doing a thorough investigation with the patient, into their whole prescription regimen and their lifestyle.

Vaccinations and Prescriptions

As you already may be aware of, a pharmacist is available to administer (i.e. inject you with) your annual flu shot. Not only does it take a load off your family doctor at a busy time of the year, but I really see it as being extremely convenient for my patients. **No prescription needed!** You can come right into the pharmacy and get your flu shot whenever you want. In addition to the flu shot, pharmacists can administer countless travel vaccines, and the list keeps growing. This is extremely convenient, especially for emergency travel situations where it can take weeks to see your family doctor. Plus, pharmacies are the places that stock the medication in the first place! The easier we can make it, the better.

When it comes to your usual prescriptions, pharmacists can renew your prescription for chronic (ongoing) conditions. Again, this makes it easier for my patients to keep their health in check and on track. (There of course are guidelines on this, in terms of the type of medications and how long one can go without seeing their physician and still remain on the same prescription.) Pharmacists may also adapt a prescription if they see necessary. In cases like this, they may suggest changing a dose or even the administration, such as providing a suspension to drink if someone can't swallow a large tablet. A conversation is of course had with a patient, and if all parties are OK with it, the pharmacy team will document the change, and it will be forwarded to their doctor so that it may be added to their patient file. This again is not only looking out for the best health of the patient, but providing some convenience to the patient and their care. Extending prescriptions is also a possibility, especially when there are extenuating circumstances and the patient may not be able to get to their doctor for a follow-up or a new prescription.

Another fantastic advantage that pharmacists have is the ability to prescribe certain medications without the diagnosis from a physician. There are two avenues when looking at this. The first is for particular things such as dealing with smoking cessation, needing an emergency oral contraceptive (morning after pill), or wanting to treat head lice. A pharmacist can have a conversation with you, create a treatment plan, and dispense the appropriate medications you need. They will then be added to your patient file and, depending on the situation, a conversation won't even need to take place with your family doctor.

The second avenue when prescribing medications is helping to relieve common health problems such as mild acne, urinary tract infections, or hemorrhoids (among many others). The degree to which a pharmacist can prescribe and help you when it comes to the medications, depends on the province/state or country in which you live. However, things are changing every year. Not only are patients feeling more taken care of and less inconvenienced, but pharmacists want to help and are at an advantage, as they are already in the community and have the medications right at their fingertips. Time can be of the essence in so many of these cases, and it feels right that pharmacists can jump in and help right away.

"Life is like a tree and its root is consciousness. Therefore, once we tend the root, the tree as a whole will be healthy."
–Deepak Chopra

Keeping It Personal

When you are managing your prescriptions or health conditions, pharmacists are at the front line with you. So it is essential to work with them and let them help you. You can think of pharmacists as having a utility belt with a collection of tools that you may not even consider, but for which may be of benefit to you and your loved ones.

Pharmacists and their teams will help demonstrate how to take your new medication. This is very helpful, especially if you are suddenly expected to take a medication that is not in the usual pill form you are used to. What if a prescription is not available in the dose prescribed? Or what if, suddenly, there is an inventory shortage for a medication? A pharmacist, especially one in a compounding pharmacy, has the knowledge and skills to compound and dispense medications so that they may be of the required dose, or even create the medication required on the spot if needed.

As the scope of practice for pharmacists expands, access to lab tests allow pharmacists to make better informed clinical decisions. Point of Care Testing (PoCT), which is done in the pharmacy, is an amazing resource to the community. It's an alternative to traditional lab testing (which can be time consuming and requires an appointment), and provides results that are current, rather than relying on results that may be weeks to months old. A great example of pharmacists having the potential to be at the forefront of diabetes prevention and management, is the HbA1c (or the A1C) test. This is a test used to detect diabetes, and it can be done quickly, with only small amounts of blood, right in the pharmacy! This makes it very accessible to the individual, and allows pharmacists to better manage their patients' diabetes. Positive changes can be made by the patient instantly, to help them become healthier much faster. Another example of PoCT can be seen in Ontario, where pharmacists have the authority to perform a procedure on tissue below the skin (e.g., collect blood by finger prick), for the purpose of chronic disease education and monitoring. I'm sure you'll agree that any time pharmacists can play a greater role in chronic disease management, everyone wins!

Something really exciting that fairly recently made its way into the field of Pharmacy is *pharmacogenomics*. Pharmacogenomics is the study of how genes affect a person's response to medication. This combines pharmacology (the science of drugs) and genomics (the study of genes and their functions) to develop effective, safe medications and doses that will be tailored to a person's genetic makeup. It can't get any more personal than that! Many drugs that are currently available to patients are "one size fits all," but they don't work the same way for everyone. It can be difficult to predict who will benefit from a medication, who will not respond at all, and who will experience negative side effects. With these new tools, we will have the ability to do that. A mentor and friend of mine, Professor John Papastergiou, along with his team, won first prize at the prestigious FIP World Congress of Pharmacy and Pharmaceutical Sciences 2016, in Buenos Aires, for his ground-breaking pharmacogenomics research project. He continues his work in this field, and it is only becoming more and more exciting. I can't wait to watch all the developments unfold in the coming years.

I have touched upon how pharmacists contribute to the lives of people every day, no matter how small or big their health concern. To mention all the contributions pharmacists make, I would need to write a whole separate book! But I feel I must now dive in to talk about the misconceptions people still have about who a pharmacist is, what they do, and how they contribute to health care on the whole. Clarity on this is valuable and empowering, no matter who you are.

Chapter Summary

- Pharmacists can assist patients with very specific services that you may not realize are available

- Managing medication profiles, administering certain vaccines and prescribing certain medications may be included

- The more you understand how a pharmacist can contribute to your health care team, the more you realize the value of your relationship with your pharmacist

- Pharmacists are with you at the front line of managing your health

Chapter 6

MISCONCEPTIONS ABOUT PHARMACISTS

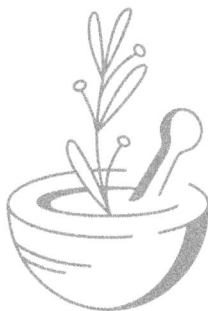

*"Details create the
big picture."*

–Sanford I. Weill

6

Contrary to what some believe, Pharmacy is an exciting and diverse career! So much more is available for a pharmacist to practice than just simply filling prescriptions. They often work alongside doctors, nurses, and other health care professionals or specialists, caring for patients and being part of their health care team. Pharmacists often conduct research that directly influences rules and regulations of various healthcare fields. They also may directly be participating in the education of future generations of pharmacists at various institutions or courses outside of the classroom.

As you can see, a pharmacist's responsibilities and work reach far beyond the prescription counter. However, many people still have huge misconceptions as to what a pharmacist actually does, and what the role in health care really entails. I know in my own life, my friends and family had a fantastic understanding as to what a pharmacist's work really is about because I was working in a pharmacy from such an early age. Only because of my own passion and dedication to the field early in my life did those around me then know that it wasn't all about just counting pills etc. I want to talk about some common misconceptions that I usually hear from people in my own community or when I meet people for the first time and tell them I am a pharmacist.

I think as with anything in life, the more you learn and understand something, the greater respect you will then have for it. Let's take a look at some of the misconceptions about pharmacists, and set the record straight.

"Pharmacists only count pills."

This is probably the first thing you think of when you think of a pharmacist: someone in a lab coat, behind the counter, counting pills, creating labels, and filling a prescription.

It is certainly how a pharmacist is portrayed in commercials and mainstream media. And of course it is what you see when you go to a pharmacy. You only see the lab coat and dozens of shelves of medications. So it makes sense for one to just assume that this is the sole role of a pharmacist.

But pharmacists do so much more! Pharmacists are constantly learning and conducting research in order to effectively educate their patients and provide counsel when it comes to their health. They are in constant communication with patients and prescribers in regard to dosing information, drug interactions, and the best course of action. When you think about it, they are a non-negotiable team member in ensuring the best care, especially when it comes to people needing life-saving medication. Pharmacists are the medication experts on a team of doctors when someone has a healthcare team. They are absolutely vital in that no other member of the team has been trained to handle this aspect of a patient's journey.

Of course, traditional "retail pharmacy" still exists and operates as usual. However, the field of Pharmacy is constantly evolving. With that evolution,pharmacists are finding a multitude of opportunities outside the pharmacy setting (which we examined previously in Chapter 4). So it is safe to say that while some certainly work in a traditional dispensary setting, pharmacists certainly do *much more* than just count pills.

"Pharmacists are only behind the scenes."

I tend to disagree with this one. In my community, I have many patients who will come to the pharmacy *first,* to talk with me before going to their physician. When a pharmacist and their team consistently show up for their patients wholeheartedly, I feel that the patient will tend to seek advice from them first, when a health issue comes up. It saves the patient a trip to the doctor, and possibly some time. As you can see, pharmacists are not just behind the scenes; they are fully at the front line of patients' health care.

Pharmacists can offer advice steeped in knowledge that connects medical conditions, lifestyles, medications, and other variables. So, of course, they are key players in one's health care team, and don't just remain behind the scenes.

The only time we would make an exception to this would be when a pharmacist is working in a lab or other sort of research facility either at a pharmaceutical company or within the government. Then of course they would be more behind the scenes when it comes to patient interaction and management. But in a general sense you can count on your pharmacist to be right there with you and for you.

"Pharmacists can never write prescriptions."

Regulations concerning writing prescriptions are highly varied across provinces, territories, states, and countries. However, when it comes down to it, pharmacists CAN prescribe medications, and it just depends on where they are located. For example, in Ontario (Canada), pharmacists can solely prescribe and dispense smoking cessation medication, as well as extending prescriptions for chronic medications in case the patient can't make it in to see their doctor.

As more regulations change, in the near future, pharmacists prescribing and dispensing medications for minor ailments, such as coughs, sore throats, pink eye, and urinary tract infections, will also be available to communities. When a pharmacist is given the authority to directly prescribe more medications, think of how well communities and the individual will be served. A patient won't have to wait to see a doctor or have to travel to see a doctor as many do when living in rural areas. How exciting for the patient and what a boost to their quality of life. Also, think of the peace of mind you would have knowing that your pharmacist may be able to help you or a family member immediately and therefore feel better sooner?

This is a reflection of putting trust in pharmacists because they deserve it. They are experts in their field and, at the end of the day, the person that most directly benefits is the patient.

"There isn't job diversity within the field of Pharmacy."

I want to change the misconception that there is not enough job diversity in the field of Pharmacy. Many seem to think there is a limited number of jobs that a pharmacist can have. This just simply isn't true! Pharmacists have many unique career paths available to them, and these paths keep expanding, thanks to the ever-changing field of healthcare. Pharmacists are members of a health care team and use evidence-based medicine when helping their team members choose the best course of medication for their patients. Did you know that pharmacists, with their associations, will actually approach legislators and take courses of action on behalf of their patient's well-being? Pharmacists are constantly involved in the research, drug development, and clinical trials of new medications. Then of course, there is always community pharmacy, which is where I have spent most of my time and effort. The possibilities for the career path of a pharmacist are truly endless!

"Pharmacists are not part of the medical team."

It is interesting to me how some people in a way disassociate pharmacists from the practice of medicine. As we have discussed, yes pharmacy originated from the making of medicines and compounds for patients. And these would have been prescribed by a physician. However, they are in no way separate. I like to think of it more in terms of being two sides of the same coin.

You have to always keep in mind: Pharmacists are THE medication experts. We are the link between a doctor's diagnosis, the prescription, and the patient. At times, we will have the final say on what the patient is being prescribed, because a pharmacist's strengths lie in combining their experience with being up to date on the most recent medication offerings and developments. When working in a hospital setting with other medical professionals, pharmacists will always add value to the medical team.

"Pharmacists can't specialize in something (like a physician)."

Many people don't realize that pharmacists have specialties. Just as with most professions, it is of benefit for a pharmacist to really hone in to something they are passionate about and develop that aspect of their work. Not only will their own work be more available, they will be of greater benefit to their patients or workplace. Just as Law is a general way describing a field of work, so is Pharmacy. The same with being a physician.

Similar to physicians, there are a wide array of specialties pharmacists can pursue, and their expertise will be different depending on their specialty. Their speciality may be a direct reflection of the community they live in and the population that surrounds them. Other times, the specialty may be a reflection of the clinic or pharmacy that they work in.

Some areas of specialty include:

- Oncology pharmacy
- Nuclear pharmacy
- Geriatric pharmacy
- Psychopharmacotherapy
- Personal pharmacy
- Nutritional support pharmacy
- Hospice pharmacy
- Pediatric pharmacy
- Poison control pharmacy

No matter what it is, trust that a pharmacist always has a specialty. If you are looking for someone specific to work with, always ask!

*"Good health is not something we can buy.
However, it can be an extremely valuable
savings account."*

−Anne Wilson Schaef

The field of Pharmacy is ever-changing and constantly presenting new opportunities for existing pharmacists or people who are looking forward to a career in pharmacy. Breakthroughs and advances in prescription medication are constantly being made, and it is up to the pharmacist to stay on top and up to date of the ever-shifting landscape. Receiving a degree in Pharmacy ("PharmD") will always guarantee you the opportunity to pursue an abundance of career pathways, as discussed in Chapter 4.

Pharmacists are known as the medication experts and, every day, the industry is creating new opportunities and unique routes to providing patients with the best healthcare services possible. A day's work as a pharmacist will always be challenging. However, you feel a sense of happiness and great accomplishment knowing that your actions directly impact those around you.

"Your body hears everything your mind says."

−Naomi Judd

As mentioned, a pharmacist is different from a physician, and both have their own unique way of approaching patients and their needs. I want to give you insight into a process of getting to know a patient and their health, which can result in some empowering results for their overall health.

Chapter Summary

- The field of pharmacy is more diverse and fulfilling then you may initially think

- There are many misconceptions that people may have towards what a pharmacist actually does, from "just counting pills" to not actually being part of the medical team on a whole

- Pharmacists are often at the forefront of providing guidance and offering advice to patients

- The field of Pharmacy is constantly evolving but one thing remains true, a Pharmacist can be thought of the medication expert on your health care team

Chapter 7

THE PROCESS OF REVERSE DIAGNOSING AND PRESCRIBING

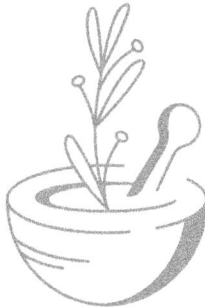

"A healthy attitude is contagious, but don't wait to catch it from others. Be a carrier."

–Tom Stoppard

7

Compared to physicians, pharmacists work a little differently when it comes to understanding a patient, their health challenges, and needs. We often use what I like to call *reverse diagnosing,* when approaching a patient's needs. I first learned this approach from both the pharmacists I worked under as a pharmacy assistant and student, and the practical training I had in school. In school we had many mock diagnosis labs where we acted the part of a pharmacist in the pharmacy lab setting and worked through different cases presented to us (both in the form of prescriptions and patients.)

When first encountering a patient and trying to gain a sense of their health challenges, pharmacists usually review the medication being prescribed. From there, we take some time with the patient to have a conversation and review their general state of health, including which medications have been prescribed and are already being taken. We can then try to determine if the medication prescribed is the most effective for what is being treated. Again, we are the experts when it comes to medication, and have a clear understanding as to how medications work, their desired and undesired effects, and any advances within the field.

This reverse diagnosing approach is of course different than when a physician approaches a patient's health. A physician will listen to a patient's concerns and complaints, create a treatment plan, and prescribe a medication. In the long run, the difference in approach to diagnosis is actually very favourable to a patient, as the same outcome is trying to be achieved via different avenues. I like to sometimes think of it as almost getting a second opinion. Often, a patient will seek out a second opinion from another physician when it comes to a health diagnosis. I feel that a pharmacist's reverse diagnosis can be the "second opinion" that a patient may need, and oftentimes without them seeking it directly.

I want to offer you a few examples of how reverse diagnosing by a pharmacist can be of benefit to a patient's health.

Example: An antibiotic prescription

A patient comes in with an antibiotic prescribed. All a pharmacist would know at this point is that the patient has an infection that requires treatment. Through questioning, the pharmacist would first find out what kind of infection is suspected or has been clinically determined. From here, assessing a patient's medication history or other relevant medical conditions and/or allergies is necessary in order to ensure that they are taking the correct medication. Now the pharmacist has clarified the nature of the condition, and ensured that the medication will be of the utmost benefit to the patient. But they won't stop there. Knowing the effects that antibiotics will have on your body, a pharmacist may then go on to recommend natural immune boosting medications, probiotics, and anything else they feel may be important to supplement the course of antibiotics, in order to replenish good gut health and prevent opportunistic infections. Opportunistic infections are infections that take advantage of the opportunity of a weakened immune system. Pharmacists can aid in preventing these types of infections in the future by helping the patient understand how to strengthen their immune system through changes to diet or taking probiotics (especially during and after taking a course of antibiotics). As you can see, when we look beyond simply what is being prescribed and why, a pharmacist can dramatically impact the future health and well-being of a patient.

Example: An anti-inflammatory prescription

A patient approaches with an anti-inflammatory prescribed. First things first: Through questioning, it is imperative to know where the pain/inflammation is, what caused it, and if it is acute (short-term) or chronic (long-term) pain. The pharmacist will then go on to investigate their past medication history, and gain an understanding of what has already been tried to reduce or alleviate pain. With their broad knowledge, the pharmacist may also suggest complementary treatments such as braces, topical options such as creams/ointments, and massage therapy. Trying to gain a broader picture of the patient's health history concerning this particular issue from the get go will save the patient time and resources in the long run. They will not be continuing on with ineffective treatments that are not working in their favor. As a pharmacist, I know that there are many more treatment options for pain and inflammation that reach far beyond a simple tablet or capsule of medication. Approaching the problem more holistically will not only treat the actual pain; it will help the patient to be in better health so that future pain may not even be an issue at all!

Not only are there topical creams and ointments that can help patients with pain or inflammation by increasing blood flow to the area in order to heal faster, patients can seek out the help of a massage therapist, chiropractor, or even have a change in physical activity in order to assist in healing. Giving the patient a basic understanding on how mental health affects our physical body, can also help and is highly beneficial as well. Studies have clearly shown that our mental health and mood will have a direct effect on physiological pain levels. It can actually be measured that our body will release more pain relieving chemicals when we experience happiness and joy, as opposed to sadness and depression. All of the above is invaluable to not only a patient's healing but future well-being and management of their symptoms.

Time and time again, we are seeing that a pharmacist's role goes way beyond just filling the prescription handed to them, or even just understanding the medication that they are prescribing. The bottom line is that more often than not, pharmacists will tend to dig deeper into a patient's case than a physician can in the short amount of time one usually spends in their office. I am not drawing any fault to this fact. Nor am I downplaying or diminishing the role of the family physician. Not at all! Physicians have been highly trained in a particular way to assess and diagnose a patient. They have different approaches and are complementary and necessary. As a pharmacist, I am lucky to have the time to take into account other details of a patient's health history, after being given a prescription to fill. This is a jumping off point for me to come to my own diagnosis (or reverse diagnosis) as I see fit, keeping in mind the best course of action for the patient in front of me.

"To keep the body in good health is a duty...
otherwise we shall not be able to keep
the mind strong and clear."

–Buddha

As I have stressed before, health care professionals should work as a team, with a patient's best interest in mind. Each has their strengths that contribute to the overall well-being of one person. When my patients tell me that they trust me more than their physician, I continuously remind them that I am a part of their health team, along with their physician. It is a collaborative effort, and I warn people to question any health care professional that is not willing to collaborate with other professionals. Usually, when someone believes they know everything, proceed with extreme caution!

I admit that there are times when I will have to further look into something foreign that is being presented to me, or will need time to find the best resource for that particular patient's case. I am never shy about this, as I want the absolute best care for those who come to me for help. My ego does not get in the way of my personal mission to provide the best care I can for those that approach me, whether they are new faces or customers I have a long-standing relationship with. No wonder my patients keep coming back and are constantly recommending their friends and family to see me! I always want what is best for them. Period.

As we have touched upon time and time again, pharmacists are much more than just a professional to fill your prescription and put some pills into a bottle. Let's look into how they are truly an advocate, or simply put, your biggest fan for your health and well-being.

Chapter Summary

- Pharmacists often use the process of reverse diagnosing when beginning the journey of helping a patient

- Reverse diagnosing begins with examining all the medications a patient is prescribed or taking then moving on to having a conversation of health challenges, investigating further in order to gain understanding to the patient's needs

- In essence, this specific approach can be seen as opposite to how a physician may approach managing a patient's health care

- At the end of the day, it is always important to remember that health professionals should work as a team with the patient's optimal health and wellbeing in mind

Chapter 8

ADVOCACY FOR PATIENTS... ADVOCACY FOR PHARMACY

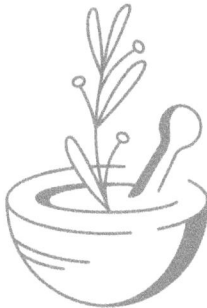

"Wherever the art of medicine is loved, there is also a love of humanity."

–Hippocrates

8

Year after year, Pharmacy changes and evolves. While this is an incredibly exciting time to be part of the profession, it can also prove to be challenging. The picture one may get of what a pharmacist does no longer exists in this day and age. As part of the vast field of health care, Pharmacy has expanded its role as part of the big picture. As we have discussed before, long gone are the days where a pharmacist simply fills a prescription at a counter. Not only are they looked upon as medication experts, pharmacists need to be recognized as integral parts of a health care team for each patient. With changes in the field constantly occurring as health care technology and research continues to evolve, it is essential that a pharmacist take on the role of **advocate** in the field of health care. Not only to advocate for our own patients and their well-being, but also to play the role of an advocate for the profession as a whole. It is a crucial part of being a pharmacist today.

Time and time again I come back to the powerful words of John F Kennedy: "If not us, who? If not now, when?" Waiting for others to take the reins when advocating for yourself and your community simply doesn't work. You have to take the lead! Being willing to take control of your life and make things happen is a necessary part of moving forward. This is an essential part of advocacy especially in your own profession. Being proactive and engaging is not only necessary, it can be highly rewarding. You and your colleagues will reap the benefits of getting out there, getting involved and getting others on board as well.

Advocacy and Patients

The relationship between a patient and a pharmacist is unique when it comes to looking at one's health care team as a whole. No matter if a patient is simply doing their yearly routines of tests and managing minor illnesses, or if they are dealing with managing chronic conditions or disease, their pharmacist plays a major role. However, it is possible that a patient really has no clear idea of what a pharmacist does, or how they are contributing to their health care picture on the whole. The future of Pharmacy everywhere is dependent on resolving this.

There are many aspects to advocating as a pharmacist to patients. First and foremost, a patient's understanding of what a pharmacist does, and all that is offered to them through this role, is critical. If a patient has a full scope of how a pharmacist fits into their health care, then they will seek out pharmacists for the help they require, and increase demand for our services. The demand for pharmacists will continue to grow, and our field will continue to expand year after year. It is therefore essential that we are thoroughly sharing all our processes with our patients, as well as the work we are putting in when it comes to treating them. Giving an insight to the patient about the processes that are part of our work will really get them on board, and possibly even excited to have us on their team. They will come to really understand all we do for them. When this happens, the respect directed toward us will level up, and the relationships with our patients will grow stronger with each interaction.

A way in which I have been able to advocate for some of my patients, is being able to speak Greek, which for many is their native language. I get so much joy when patients are referred to me because they were told by a current patient that I speak their language. For example, one Greek patient was tired of staff at the previous pharmacy he went to, constantly changing and not being able to communicate with him in a clear and understanding manner. When he came to my pharmacy (through a referral), he had such a sigh of relief! I went over all his medications with him, spoke to his doctor, and recommended to stop medications no longer needed. I packaged his medications in weekly pill packs because it helped him stay more organized, and I even wrote in Greek how and when to take his medications. He was so grateful, as was I. He felt empowered and taken care of, and I felt that I was truly contributing to his overall well-being, as we could talk about his health in his native tongue. Experiences like this require a little more effort and compassion on my end, but truly are the most rewarding!

"If you think wellness is expensive, try illness."
–Unknown

Advocacy and Promotion

Let's examine what advocacy looks like if you are a practicing pharmacist or are on your way to becoming one. When looking to shine a light on Pharmacy and what you have to offer as a pharmacist, I suggest you start with the neighborhood you are based in first. Focusing on community is an obvious way to engage potential patients. However, when you engage with your community and are prepared to educate them on Pharmacy and its role in the health care system, you are also advocating on behalf of the whole field. It is essential to remember that you are part of a bigger picture. Even though many of us can end up working alone as pharmacists, we have to always keep in mind that in fact we are part of a larger team, and that team consists of all pharmacists in the field. Imagine if all pharmacists practiced this?! The respect and growth of our jobs would grow exponentially.

Keep an eye out for opportunities to be involved in your community. Perhaps you can give a talk at a wellness center, or seek out a way to get involved with a local school. Sure, some of these opportunities can take us out of our comfort zone, and may not have immediate financial returns, but you have to remember that these actions are always part of the bigger picture of growing not only your practice but the practice of Pharmacy as a whole. Coming from behind the counter, and creating face-to-face connections with people in your neighborhood and surrounding community, is an easy and inspiring way to advocate.

A wonderful example of how I have personally connected with my community is when I was donating bandages, wrist/back braces, gauze, and a few more self-care items, at a community drop-in center for those less fortunate in the area. The exceptional people that work and volunteer at the center quickly began to recognize me when I would go in to drop off a donation, and soon I didn't even have to introduce myself. I developed a personal relationship with them. (Some even became my patients!) One day, shortly after I dropped some items off, I was at my pharmacy, working away, when someone who worked at the center came by to ask me if I could come over and give a presentation to those who would drop in during the day. Even before asking what they would want me to talk about, I wholeheartedly agreed! I felt honored to have been asked, and for the opportunity to be even more involved. The drop-in center was so grateful for my donations, and told me I could talk about anything I wanted. This is a prime example of how a simple gesture of donating in your community can lead to many great things, personally and professionally.

Year after year, pharmacists are moving from traditional dispensing roles to more patient-centered services. This is no longer just the future of our field, but already becoming the norm right now! It is an inspiring time to be a pharmacist, as we will actually be part of moulding the future of the field. However, in order to do this, we as individuals must be dedicated to advocating for the profession on all fronts and in all capacities. I will continue to ensure that people know about this wonderful field and all the possibilities for health care that it holds. But advocacy has more of an impact when there is a whole group of people standing up and speaking about something. The power of the collective is immense. Advocating for the field of Pharmacy will allow it to continue to change and flourish over time. It is so critical to educate people in order to make sure advances we as pharmacists have had in the field continue to be highlighted and celebrated. It especially sets us up to continue to be a non-negotiable aspect when looking at the field of health care as a whole.If you are a pharmacist, I hope you will join me!

We have to always remember that Pharmacy has the power to actually change someone's life. Let's put all the pieces together of what we have been discussing, and remember how each action and conversation is integral to the bigger picture at hand.

Chapter Summary

- Pharmacists must be viewed as integral parts of any health care team

- Advocacy within the profession is essential in order to keep the profession at the forefront of conversations within the industry and community at large

- Pharmacists must also be willing to be advocates for their patients so that the patient may receive the best care possible

- Patient-centered services are not only becoming the norm but are the future for the field of Pharmacy

Chapter 9

PUTTING ALL THE PIECES TOGETHER

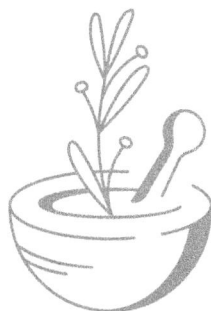

"The first wealth is health."

–Ralph Waldo Emerson

9

We have examined many aspects of why Pharmacy is an essential part of healthcare and people's lives as a whole. I like to think of the pharmacist's role, in the large puzzle of people's health plans, as a sort of center point where many things will come to light and be filtered through. Since pharmacists strive to have the most up-to-date and evidence-based knowledge surrounding medications and the conditions or ailments that are treated with them, we can act as this sort of gathering place of knowledge and people. At the end of the day, pharmacists have the power and vision to put all the pieces together for our patients, so that they are not left to have to do that themselves. They can look to their pharmacist to do that heavy lifting, and trust in a path to greater health when we are directly involved. I can hear a collective sigh of relief already...

Health Care Professionals Come Together to Help the Patient

It is imperative that we understand and always remember that each health care professional has their own education and work in their respective fields. Each field is designed to help patients in a very specific way, and be a specialized part of one's health care team. As pharmacists, not only can we be seen as individuals in that we have a specific role to play in the larger picture, we also can act as this sort of middle ground, where everyone's contributions can meet. Pharmacists can aid in understanding what the objective is, and create a snapshot in an effort to effectively help our patients. Since it is a pharmacist's field of expertise, when it comes down to one's medications, we want to attempt to navigate any and all recommendations put forth. Let's do a brief overview of where a medication suggestion may start, and how it leads to administration.

A specialist may offer a patient their first real diagnosis and recommendation of a plan of care. With this plan of care may certainly come suggestions for particular medications to assist in managing their condition or concern. A patient will then follow up with their family doctor. The doctor will then weigh in on the specialist's findings, and further solidify a plan of care based on their knowledge and the patient's health history. A specialist or family doctor may write the patient's prescription that they will bring to the pharmacy or have administered at the hospital. If a patient is being hospitalized or receiving at-home care, it will be a nurse or a nursing aid who will be in charge of administering medication and highlighting the practicality of it to the patient. However, whenever there is a prescription involved, there must also be a willingness of the patient to actually take the medication and want to improve their health. No matter if the condition is urgent or not, the final piece is always the compliance of the patient and accepting the prescription. One definitive example of this is when someone receives a prescription to help them stop smoking. If they haven't made a conscious decision to really quit, the medication will only do so much. They have to want to quit and be willing to receive help.

"It is part of the cure to want to be cured."

–Seneca

Managing the Details

Another aspect of being a center point of putting all the pieces of a health care plan together, is being up to date with a patient's medical history and personal details so that a pharmacist can provide them guidance in making choices that suit them. This includes personal preferences and values. As a pharmacist, you may facilitate a negotiating ground, remembering that this is not only about the patient's well-being physically, but mentally and spiritually as well.

For example, someone may subscribe to a faith that teaches that a woman shouldn't have an abortion. Unfortunately, in this case, I have some patients who have been prescribed a birth control pill and feel uneasy about taking it, as they think the pill has something to do with aborting a pregnancy. I go on to educate them that one of the birth control uses is to *prevent* pregnancy, not *abort* it. We would then go on to discuss how birth control is used for a variety of conditions, and is also a popular and effective option for managing and treating hormonal imbalances that may cause symptoms such as painful periods and acne. As a pharmacist, you have to be ready to have these types of discussions with your patients, to make sure they are properly informed to make the best decisions for their health. Too many times, people seek out advice from individuals for topics they have no expertise in, and this is when misinformation and confusion can occur.

You can also be mindful of such things as a patient's personal choices and values when it comes to their lifestyle. I have encountered some patients who are strict vegans and will not ingest medications with gelatin coating. Or patients who have concerns regarding the packaging of their medications, and want to ensure that as much of it as possible is recyclable and not just going straight to a landfill. I take pride in being conscious of what packaging I use at my pharmacy. I try to do what I can with what is available to me. For example, when organizing patients' medications and vitamins, the weekly pill packages I use are 100% recyclable. Even though it comes at a higher cost to my pharmacy than other packaging options, it is my way of doing my part in keeping our green planet green. Thankfully, many patients share that same point of view and really appreciate it. At the same time, my patients' health comes first, and when a request of theirs can interfere with the high standards of dispensing that I practice with, that is where I explain myself so that they clearly understand. For example, a patient wanted to reuse the same vial I previously filled their medication in. I explained to them that even though I understood they wanted to leave a smaller carbon footprint, unfortunately the vial was no longer sterile and wouldn't be safe to reuse. (Think about it: That vial would have been touched at least 90 times if it contained 3-months' worth of medication, and if the medication was to be taken 2 to 3 times a day, you would be looking at that vial being touched at least 270 times in that same 3-month window.) As long as I educate my patients when a concern is brought up, we always come to a result that both of us can agree on. It's all about listening to their concerns and then educating them on my professional point of view.

It comes down to being prepared and being mindful. Sometimes the process of filling a prescription, delivering a medication into a patient's hand, and getting them to implement it into their lives, is not as straightforward as it seems. We have to remain open minded and compassionate to *everyone's* needs.

Navigating the Media and the Internet

Many of us are guilty of using "Dr. Google" to self-diagnose or to do research on our conditions, concerns, medications, etc. While the internet can certainly be a tool of self-empowerment, it can also lead to many misunderstandings. We all have to remember that it is only ever a snapshot of information, and does not take the place of speaking to someone directly, who may have 10 to 15 (or even more!) years' experience on the matter. I always urge not only my patients, but my family and friends as well, to seek direct advice from their pharmacist. A great example that we are very familiar with is when the internet lists "home remedies" for something, but they have no evidence of working, and can actually harm you. Please remember that anyone can post online and sound pretty convincing if they use a professional title and leave a comment in a blog. Chances are that you have come across this yourself, but did you take the time to see if this "professional" has a license, is registered with their respective college, in good standing and allowed to practice? Just be careful!

> *"You can't control what goes on outside, but you CAN control what goes on inside."*
>
> –Wayne Dyer

This also applies to when articles are published online through different media outlets. I think we have to remain very discerning when reading articles online about the medical and pharmaceutical industry. With things constantly changing and ever evolving, we have to remain mindful and objective when reading about developments. As a pharmacist, I will always dig deeper so that I may not only educate myself but also be able to talk about things with my patients if they so happen to be brought up.

I will never forget an example that came up not too long ago. I noticed that people kept reposting a news story that focused on a drug that allegedly cured cancer and only cost pennies to make. But "Big Pharma" wasn't interested in it because the profits would not be there. As you can imagine, it did not take long for this sort of story to go viral, and for there to be a lot of public outcries. I immediately began doing some further research online into this particular study. It only took a few minutes to discover the whole story: that while the drug cured particular cancers in mice, it actually *caused* other cancers in mice! I couldn't imagine the public outrage and lawsuits if the drug was actually used to treat cancer and began negatively impacting people's health. It took me only two extra minutes to find out this necessary piece of information to the story, which many would not think to dig deeper into. But bottom line, this is my job. And I want to bring my expertise to my clients and patients so that they may be educated and make the right decisions for themselves.

Avoiding Serious Drug Interactions

Many people are taking several medications daily. This is a very normal occurrence, especially when dealing with patients who are suffering from multiple conditions. Organizing them into when you should be taking some at certain times of the day, is one thing. However, avoiding taking certain medications together can result in major complications. It could even lead to a life or death situation. Someone might have read or been told that two medications interact, and from experience, we as pharmacists know that it isn't necessarily an interaction that the patient has to worry about. It is a fact that they actually require both medications. Sometimes it is as easy as taking the two medications a couple of hours apart. Another example is when the absorption of one medication might decrease when taken with another one. That being said, if a patient won't remember to take the second medication at a later time, one recommendation to them could be to continue taking the medications together. Some absorption is better than not taking the medication at all (depending on the specific case that presents itself, of course).

As a pharmacist, it is one of my great responsibilities to have a clear record and understanding of my patients' health histories and the medications they are taking or have taken. Avoiding having serious drug interactions is crucial. This not only includes combining different prescription drugs but also combining prescription drugs with over- the-counter medications. It is imperative, as a pharmacist, that I dive deep and do a thorough investigation as to all the possible medications my patient has or will be taking. Even asking about simple things like basic cold or pain medications, may save someone a trip to the emergency room.

Looking Ahead to the Future

"The doctor of the future will give no medicine but will interest his patients in the care of the human frame, in diet and in the cause and prevention of disease."

–Thomas Edison

Thomas Edison's above quote is one that really makes you think. When we look ahead to the future of healthcare in general, the health of the individual will extend beyond just seeing their physician for a prescription and then going to their pharmacist to get it filled and perhaps some further guidance as well. The rise in a more holistic approach to medicine and care is already evident.

Naturopathic doctors are just now beginning to receive the recognition they deserve in health care. This is not surprising, as an increased interest in alternatives to "traditional" medicine has been seen over recent years. More and more people are looking to holistic medicine for its focus on giving the opportunity for the body to heal itself, through focusing on balancing the body, mind, and spirit. Practices such as acupuncture, biofeedback, faith healing, folk medicine, meditation, vitamin therapy, and even fasting, are becoming more mainstream and can now be seen as definite options when looking to alternative therapies in healing. Alternative and natural therapies should definitely not be overlooked when looking to complement one's health. It is becoming very clear that the patient will benefit most when traditional and alternative forms of medicine are combined and tailored to the individual needs.

"I have chosen to be happy because it is good for my health."
–Voltaire

Where does Pharmacy come into play in this future landscape of healthcare? As pharmacists, we help people to take charge of their own health. King Solomon said, *"As he thinketh in his heart, so is he."* This quote aims to remind us that the individual holds the key to every condition, good or bad, that enters into their life, and by working patiently and intelligently upon their thoughts, they transform themselves. Researchers are showing measurable evidence of the power of one's thoughts and mindset, in medical studies conducted using placebos. Placebos (which are an inert substance, therefore having no therapeutic value on a patient), when used in place of actual medication, are actually being shown to create positive results in patients' health. This is a prime example of the power of one's thoughts. When it comes down to it, there is scientific proof that one's health is directly affected by their thoughts alone. Pharmacists are already shifting toward more service and counselling-based practices, and shifting a focus to more preventative, medicine-based approaches with their patients.

In order to be a great pharmacist, you of course have to be well-educated and understand your role in the health care world. But it's much more than that. A *great* pharmacist is someone who is willing to take the time to listen and go above and beyond for their patients. It's the little things that, while they may take more time in the present, will bring you greater rewards in the long run.

Chapter Summary

- A pharmacist can be the center of one's plan of care; a focal point where many things can be brought to light and understood

- No matter what the circumstance, it will always come down to the patient's willingness to follow through with a course of action to benefit their health, whether that involves medication or not

- Pharmacists can manage the details for a patient's plan of care and present it to them in a comprehensible manner

- One should always seek advice directly from a pharmacist: do not rely on "Dr. Google"

- It is imperative that pharmacists have a clear understanding on a patient's health history so that they can prevent negative drug interactions

- The future of healthcare is moving towards a more holistic lens and will likely involve many different practitioners including naturopathic doctors, acupuncturists and other alternative and natural therapies

- One's thoughts play a large role in their overall health: keeping them positive is essential

Chapter 10

CHANGING LIVES ONE CONVERSATION AT A TIME

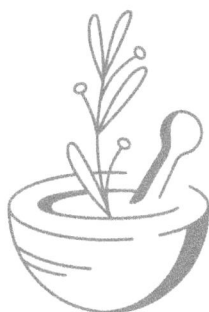

"You never know when a moment and a few sincere words can have an impact on a life."

–Zig Ziglar

10

In October of 2017, I decided to open my own pharmacy. It was clear to me that I wanted to run my own practice, create my own community health hub, and help people one-on-one. Other aspects of the field were exciting, but what drew me to Pharmacy in the first place was working with patients face to face. Located in downtown Toronto, I invited in many different people from all walks of life. As I quickly learned, every single person's needs can be different, and this certainly keeps me on my toes.

YouTube sensation, entrepreneur and personal growth mentor Evan Carmichael sums up how my life has changed by changing other people's lives: "Your purpose comes from your pain. If you don't know what your purpose is, think about the most painful moments in your life. Your purpose is to serve others who are going through that same pain." As I help relieve pain and obstacles in people's lives, it helps me grow and defeat my own pains and obstacles. Carmichael talks about how when you find your purpose, it will fuel you for life. He goes on to say that your purpose is your source of power. That is what I have discovered as I serve others in my practice and has changed me for the better. I truly feel that being of service to my community through being a great pharmacist and operating my own health hub has helped me gain that sense of personal power and strength. This then extends beyond the walls of my practice to my personal life and really to the community on a whole.

Everyone is invited to have conversations with my staff and me: **No prescription needed!** Sometimes a conversation that may actually change someone's life will start with a simple question like "Where are the bandages?" or "How can I stop this runny nose?" I find that if you are willing to take the time and listen to people, you will discover so much more about what is going on with their health as a whole. After just a few minutes of my undivided attention, they will receive exactly what they need, and none of what they don't. Of course, my short-term sales suffer. I have actually steered people away from purchases because I knew that they didn't really need the product or over-the-counter medication they were originally seeking. However, what I have definitely noticed is that my practice continues to thrive because of the relationships I am creating with my patients and clients. They can see and feel that I am genuinely interested in their total well-being; and because of that, I grow relationships, not just profits.

"Every negative belief weakens the partnership between mind and body."
–Deepak Chopra

Being honest with anyone who walks through the door seeking advice or an opinion is extremely important to me.

My patients ask me for advice about their health in general, and sometimes on topics that have nothing to do with Pharmacy because they know I simply won't feed them a bunch of invaluable information or lies. If I cannot provide a well-informed and honest answer in regard to a patient's inquiry, I simply say, "I don't know enough about that." But the conversation does not end there. I will go ahead and do more research and look further into the topic at hand. I usually learn something new myself that I can then pass on to future patients with the same inquiry, or I refer them to someone who can directly help them. I never see this as a missed opportunity for my practice. Every interaction is a possibility for a long-term relationship, where I can then become the person they will come to with future concerns and questions, thus earning their loyalty and keeping their trust in the long run. A relationship with a patient is all built on trust and effective communication. When those key factors are in place, you will find that your practice grows, all the while making a real difference in people's lives and your community.

Medications are a wonderful way to help people lead healthier and happier lives, but only when they are prescribed and used properly. Some people don't really want to be taking medications at all, and I don't blame them! Sometimes medications can be a burden on our day-to-day lives, especially when they require that we take them at specific times under specific conditions, while trying to avoid interactions and unwanted side effects. Medications can make people happier and healthier in the short term (e.g., when we are dealing with a cold or flu), or long term (e.g., when treating things such as an autoimmune disease or psoriasis). However, I have encountered many cases where people stay on medication longer than they should, for a variety of reasons. Sometimes communication has not been clear enough between the prescribing specialist, the family doctor, and the original pharmacist dispensing the medication. The patient then is simply worried that if they were to stop their medication, their symptoms may return. This results in a patient's quality of life being affected, and may also result in minor to major health complications. I like to work on the possibility of "deprescribing" medications with my patients. This requires more work on my part for sure, but if I can actually change someone's life for the better, it far outweighs the time invested. It all starts with conversations regarding medications they are taking, why they were prescribed in the first place, and eventually leads to discussions about other contributing factors to their health, such as diet and exercise. During this process, I always remain available and just a visit or phone call away to support them (**No prescription needed** to connect with me!).

The smile on someone's face, when they stop a medication they no longer need, puts an even bigger smile on my face. It is like handcuffs are being taken off the individual. They no longer have to stop in the middle of a meal just to take medication with food, or postpone a snack because they have to take something on an empty stomach to have it better absorbed. They gain so much more freedom and less stress in their lives. Many times, a patient will be so excited and motivated after I have helped them stop a medication, that they start changing other aspects of their lifestyle, like diet and exercise, and they can't wait to continue investigating if there is a possibility of stopping another medication. I become just as excited because I am directly helping someone change their lives for the better. I can see a clear chain reaction that happens with these particular patients as well. Soon enough, I will begin meeting patients' family and friends, as they are so inspired by the transformation in their friend or loved one, they want the same for themselves.

This is the heart of my practice. Time and time again, I watch patients grow into more happy and healthy individuals because I have taken the time to listen, and have the willingness to help and invest in them. I'm so grateful that I have truly created a health and wellness hub at my pharmacy, and am known for providing more than what one may expect from a pharmacist. I hope that I may shine a light on this way of running a Pharmacy practice to many, in order to not only bring change to communities, but to also create excitement around an important but possibly overlooked profession.

"To ensure good health: eat lightly,
breathe deeply, live moderately, cultivate
cheerfulness, and maintain an interest in life."
−William Londen

No Prescription Needed...

I'm sure that when you began reading this book, you thought you had a strong understanding of how a pharmacist fits into your idea of health care for yourself and your loved ones. However, I am sure I surprised you with revealing some new and exciting perspectives, not only on the field of Pharmacy but also how a pharmacist can help you. As I said before, at the end of the day, the role of a pharmacist is so much more than standing behind a counter and filling out a prescription. It is about advocating for health care in the community and beyond! I urge you to get more involved with your pharmacist and advocate for yourself and your health. If you want to lead a healthier life filled with more vitality and energy, I bet your pharmacist can assist you in starting that journey.

If you are a student or have just started your role as a pharmacist, I hope this book opened your mind to all the ways you can be involved in the healthcare industry. Really take time to focus on your passions and continue to explore how those passions can feed into different opportunities for you. As we have discussed the field is constantly growing and evolving. Now is the time to really go after what you want or advocate for our field in your community. The only way to go is up!

I look forward to a future where a pharmacist *always* works hand in hand with their patient, toward their best and most healthy life. My passion for my community continues to grow as my practice grows, and I look forward to helping more pharmacists take the step to developing a more patient-centered and elevated practice. The possibility of a pharmacist being an integral and respected part of each community is within reach. When it comes down to it, it again is about the patient and their health. We only have so many years to live. Why not live them in the best health you can so that you may achieve your goals and contribute to your community and the lives of those around you?

I encourage you to get to know your pharmacist. If you don't feel comfortable talking or relating to your current pharmacist, find one that you do! We all have our strengths and it will be worth it to find a pharmacist for you and your family that provides individualized attention and personalized care. Think of your pharmacist as part of your health care team. You have your doctor, dentist, and ophthalmologist, and you may even have a massage therapist or physiotherapist as well. These people keep you living your best life year after year. Get your pharmacist on board with this team (especially when managing chronic illness, or better yet, to prevent them!). You will not look back when you begin to understand the value of your pharmacist to your overall health. They will become your closest health ally!

"Prevention is better than cure."
–Desiderius Erasmus

It has been such a pleasure sharing this book. I also look forward to meeting you. Yes, you! If you have any questions or are just in the neighborhood, never hesitate to stop by for a chat... *no prescription needed!*

www.No**Prescription**Needed**Book**.com

ABOUT THE AUTHOR

Born and raised in Toronto, ON (Canada), Dr. George Frangias attended the University of Toronto and then went south of the border to continue his education. He is a graduate of the Massachusetts College of Pharmacy and Health Sciences (MCPHS), in Boston, MA (USA), where he earned his Doctorate in Pharmacy, in 2012. Upon graduation, George worked at multiple independent pharmacies, allowing him to stay in more intimate settings where he got to develop relationships with his patients on a personal level. This led to him acquiring his own pharmacy in downtown Toronto, in 2017, to continue practicing where he can maintain personal relationships with not only his patients but his staff as well.

He is an active member of the Ontario Pharmacists Association and the Canadian Pharmacists Association, to name a couple, where he continues to develop himself professionally, and participates in advocating for Pharmacy and his patients as well.

George strongly believes that the accessibility of the community pharmacist is essential when it comes to actively screening and monitoring patients for various acute and chronic diseases. He credits the advancements in his practice, and his willingness to strengthen his personal connection to his patients, as being largely due to his commitment to continued personal development. This is his first book.

www.No**Prescription**Needed**Book**.com

TESTIMONIALS

George and his team are a gift to the community! The environment in his pharmacy is warm and welcoming, no matter what time it is, or how busy it is. I can see that all his employees take great pride in their work, and I always have a personal experience. I wouldn't trust anyone else when it comes to managing my family's health concerns and plan of care.

—**George Michailidis,**
Entrepreneur

Year after year, George has shown himself to be a true leader in pharmacy. His passion for his work shines, and is evident in everything he does. Whether it be managing his pharmacy business, teaching the next generation or helping in the community, George is a true example of how a pharmacist is an integral part of any health care team!

—**Dr. John Metyas,**
PharmD, RPH

George treats everyone like family! So refreshing in these times when more and more people seem disconnected from one another.

**—Mani Taghaboni,
Pharmaceutical Industry**

Over the years I have worked with George in and out of the pharmacy setting. His enthusiasm for his work and life in general is contagious. He advocates for his profession in a way that I have not seen for years. The younger generation of pharmacists is lucky to have him as their mentor.

**—Mark Merkouris,
Musician & Artist**

I had no idea how much my pharmacist played a role in my overall wellbeing until I met George! He goes above and beyond, time and time again. With George's help my health is back on track. My body and spirit haven't felt this good in YEARS! Thanks George!

**—Evangelina Sirmis,
Artist & Grateful Patient**

www.ingramcontent.com/pod-product-compliance
Lightning Source LLC
Chambersburg PA
CBHW060617210326
41520CB00010B/1367